C000264058

Natasha Jones

MANDEMIC

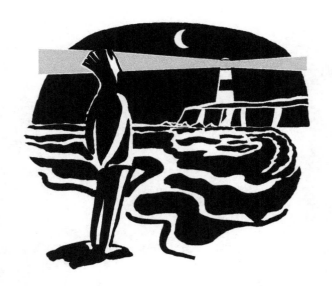

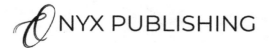

ONYX PUBLISHING

First published in 2021 by Onyx Publishing, an imprint of
Notebook Publishing of Notebook Group Limited,
20–22 Wenlock Road,
London, N1 7GU.

www.notebookpublishing.com

ISBN: 9781913206567

A CIP catalogue record for this book is available
from the British Library.

Typeset by Notebook Group Limited.

To my son, who is the most courageous male I have had the privilege of spending time with.

To my daughter: may you find true love with a man whose role models have shown him the light of conscious masculinity, allowing him to openly adore both your inner and outer strength and beauty.

Thank you, Ron, for believing in myself and the Man; for transporting this story from my mind onto paper with each of your inspirational drawings.

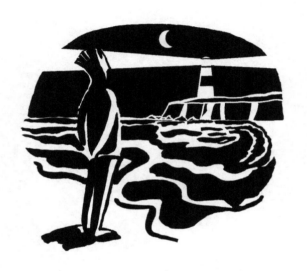

FOREWORD

AS I SAT QUIETLY in the midst of Spring 2020 with the pandemic of COVID-19, it dawned on me that a bigger pandemic had been at play for some time: the bashing of the male, if you will. Let's call it a Mandemic.

I was called to be a lawyer to help others, which followed my study of human nature in psychology and my fulfilling of a lifelong intrigue in what makes people 'tick'.

The necessity to exist in the masculine energy of success, driven and defined by disciplined focus on planning and tangible results, was the way many of us were taught to build a thriving law practice in the late nineties. For over twenty years, I observed those who I both worked alongside, socialised with, and acted on behalf of, in what was typically described and viewed as a 'Man's World' of Law and Business.

Observing the terrible effect that life-changing events—redundancy (in my work); loss of young parents, children, and marriages (in my personal life)—I began to more clearly and closely see and recognise the struggle of grieving and coming to terms with the 'rug being pulled out from under' a person. Increasingly, I empathised with individuals—typically men—who seemed to never allow themselves to develop self-love/nurturing skills. I began a journey of passion to inspire resilience and help them (i.e., clients, friends, and husbands of friends) find the tools to cope with the devastating events in their lives.

Men working in a man's world who have found professional success are often unable to share their feelings and emotions, and so deal with (and ultimately deny) these alone.

I felt that I was able to meet them where they were, as I fully understood the environment and position they were in, having lived it myself, and so I became uniquely placed to help and be a trusted advisor.

I dearly hope that the world can catch these people and show them that, when they fall (as most of us do), they can be held and nurtured, and are allowed to protect and sustain themselves while they re-find their balance. I hope that they can find a catalyst for change, and see that what might feel like the worst thing to have ever happened can actually become the best opportunity.

The Samaritans report that the highest suicide rate in the UK is amongst males aged between forty-five and forty-nine years, and there are so many out there—and they are suffering alone.

One, some, or all thirty-two of the good habits detailed in this book—all of which I passionately believe in—can make a difference and set a struggling person on a new path to finding new solutions and new pathways that will work for them. It is a taster; tempting a person to take their first step of a journey of a thousand (or more) miles, which might be concerned with finding the energy, hope, and enthusiasm experienced in their youth.

Many clients, I am sure, will attest to the fact that I regularly refer to my belief that 'male' and 'female' are two sides of a perfect coin. It is my belief that working collectively together with a joint beneficial focus is the best way forward. I am not a fan of division, finger-pointing, or point-scoring by 'either' sex, whether it be in the workplace, the home, or society as a whole.

I have been fortunate to have had some fantastic male role models and mentors; my perfect blend is a new hybrid combination of traditional stoicism with a dash of self-care and a sprinkling of emotional openness. As a mother, I hope that my children, their peers, and my unborn grandchildren can all learn to find a way to both applaud and nurture masculinity. In my role as a daughter, I see now that I was very fortunate to be raised in a family where support and praise were given for all achievements; where listening was valued; and in which kindness and pulling together was a simple but mandatory family (and extended family) mantra—come what may. **#Gratitude**.

INTRODUCTION

ONCE UPON A TIME, in a land far away, across seven seas, existed a man who had lived for more than four decades. In his youth, the man had excitedly planned his life with hope and enthusiasm. He had dreamed of having a family of his own, a home he was proud of, and a career in which he was successful and well-liked. He took for granted that he would be fit and healthy, happy, and loved by many when he 'got there'—the proverbial 'destination'.

One day, a pandemic, from which many had died, reached the man's land, and he was told he should stay at home and must not leave. The man was scared and angry, and, for thirty-two days, he listened to the news—which, every day, talked about death and the thousands of people losing their lives to the pandemic. He sat in his house day after day, thinking of every person who had upset him and blaming every event and every occasion that had not worked for his benefit. He projected his frustration onto others, deciding they were to blame for his misery. As each day passed by, he began to reflect upon his life and began to see the walls of his house and the people whom he loved and lived with differently. He began to realise that he could no longer blame travelling to work, or the traffic, or the people he worked with, for his bad moods. He began to accept that, for many years, he had lived a joyless, miserable life, and had lost his drive and energy for living: his mojo; his spark.

As time went on, to the man's horror, he could see that he had not been very nice for longer than he cared to remember—not only to those he cared for, but pretty much everyone: those he spoke to in shops; on the street; who he worked with; anyone, in fact, he had interacted with. He was ashamed to admit that he had not shown heartfelt thanks to anyone for a long, long time. He realised that he had long ago stopped being kind, compassionate, and considerate. In fact, he had existed for such a long time in his own miserable world that he didn't really see or consider other people, especially his children, parents, and siblings. He believed they were important to him, but he had never quite found the time to give them his full attention, show them love and affection, or pay full attention when he was with them. He realised, with sadness, that he did not really listen when others spoke; his mind would simply drift off somewhere else. He often considered that he was too busy, in a bad mood, or too tired, and had so often responded with 'not now' that many had stopped seeking his attention, leaving him to dwell on his perceived troubles. He would drink alcohol, thinking it would cheer him up, telling himself he liked the taste, but the following day, he would feel even more hopeless, short-tempered, and grumpy than before.

With realisation settling in, the man went to bed feeling miserable. As always, he scrolled social media on his phone. He carried his phone with him all the time; it was the first thing he looked at every morning and the last thing each night. He looked to see what other people were up to, which, more often than not, agitated him further. Everyone else seemed to be so happy— everyone except for him. The men he had known when he was younger had better houses, better cars, and went on better holidays than he did, and so his resentment grew. Deep down, he acknowledged how easy it was to nosily look in on other people's lives, but that it took far more effort to actively engage in and live his own. Focusing on others as a distraction was easier and far more comfortable than looking inwards at himself and his own life.

He lay in bed, as he did every night, feeling annoyed. His body was exhausted, but he couldn't go to sleep believing that, yet again tomorrow, he would be tired and the day would again feel difficult and dreary. He began to realise that he didn't really live his life but merely existed from day to day. Years later, he was never sure whether he had drifted off to sleep or whether he had just begun to think differently. He began to acknowledge that he had, for as long as he could remember, looked for reasons to be offended. Over time, his mind had become closed but attached to everything. He had asked himself for years, 'Is this it?' and he had stopped hoping and dreaming, everything feeling like too much effort. His mind was full of so much resentment that it had no space or energy to even look for hope or joy. A voice often loudly interrupted his thoughts at inconvenient times or when he was alone—and especially in bed—taking him back to past actions and causing him to feel regret or catapulting him to a future that terrified him. The thought of failing or being rejected was so terrifying he had stopped trying anything—and the realisation hit hard.

The man realised he no longer intentionally moved his body; he always felt too tired, and for more than a decade had made so many excuses he was no longer disciplined enough to make the effort to regularly exercise. Yet as a young man, he had exercised several times a week and enjoyed playing sports until he was physically exhausted. With a wry smile, he proudly acknowledged that he had been a fine sportsman. Back then, despite being physically tired, his mind always seemed to be clear, and he had felt energised and hopeful. For so long, a berating voice had either criticised failures of his past or generated fear for his future, so much so that he no longer felt able to decisively take action unless forced to do it.

Deep, deep down, somewhere far down in the man's stomach, he felt a flutter of—what was it? Was it a tiny hint of excitement? Was it the same feeling he had felt often as a young man? Or was he starting to dream? Then, the feeling quickly faded away. It had been a long, long time since he had felt anything at all, let alone a hint of hope or flutter of excitement. The man acknowledged that he rarely finished anything off, as most of the time, he felt too tired. People around him irritated him by trying to hurry him along. Why could they not understand that he did things in his way and in his own time? So what if he was slow? He felt another flutter. It had been so long since he had made even a plan, let alone finished a task. Then, with a jolt, he realised he had judged everyone around him. This was because he had told himself that it was 'okay for them' as 'their lives were easy' and 'they did not know what it felt like to be unproductive and like him; empty and dead inside, walking through life as a ghost'. For once, the loud voice did not agree or rant about life being unfair; instead, there was just silence. The man's body was still, and he noticed every breath in and back out again. *Ba boom. Ba boom.* The beating of his heart.

A sound diverted his attention; not a frightening sound, but a comforting and almost familiar sound. He looked into the dark, trying hard to adjust his eyes and peering harder as a vague outline of a lighthouse appeared in the distance. He could hear the sound of waves softly lapping against the foot of the cliff upon which the lighthouse stood proud, a beam of light reflecting onto the rippling water.

A few minutes passed and the man felt calm. What was this feeling? It felt almost warm and soft inside; it felt nice. This was not what he was used to. Where was the berating voice? Again, he was 'feeling' something; an alien experience which he was certainly not used to. From the lighthouse came a gentle voice and, as it spoke, the light of the lighthouse glowed brighter. 'Why do you choose to live like this,

Man?' The man lay still—there were no words to say. Once again, he felt the beating of his heart. *Ba boom. Ba boom.* Again, the lighthouse glowed brightly. 'You had such hope, optimism, and energy in your youth. Why will you not now allow yourself to live again and to be happy, Man?'

As the man was about to repeat in his angry voice his usual rant of blaming everyone else, describing how harsh the cards that life had dealt him had been and rebuffing with a statement that 'it was just the way he was', deep in his belly, a gentle quivering voice spoke, silencing the berating voice:

'Help me. I am the soul of this man, but I don't know where to start because the berating voice always talks over me.'

The lighthouse gently soothed, 'I will help you, but I am only a lighthouse. I will shine my light, but you have to save yourself.'

There was silence for a few moments. 'Man, do you want to do this?'

'Yes,' said the soul of the man.

'Okay,' said the lighthouse, 'I will shine thirty-two times. Pay attention, as each evening,

I will illuminate a word for you to consider and adopt in relation to new habits that can help you. Do you think you can you do this, Man?'

The man nodded in the dark.

The lighthouse commanded, 'Each morning when you wake, you will say the words out loud: "My life is my own". And each day, you must focus on your daily habit to the fullest extent that you are able to.'

'I will,' agreed the man.

And this is how the man began to form new habits and changed his life for the better, forever.

HABITS

Habitus: Custom, Tradition, Practice, **Habit.**

Motivation is what gets you started, but habits are what keep you going. Challenge yourself, but remember to be patient, as it might take forty days to form or break a habit—and perhaps one thousand days until mastered. Set goals that are realistic and take small steps. What good habits do you pledge, today to begin? **#Habit**

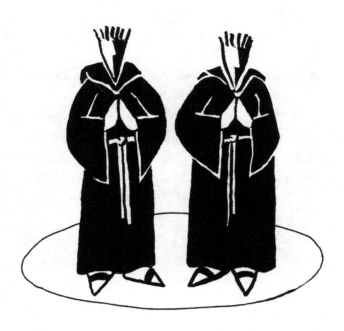

LISTEN

Ausculto: Hear, Obey, Apply the Ears, **Listen.**

As Mother Nature gave us two ears to listen with and only one mouth to speak with, perhaps listen to hear rather listen to respond. Can you speak less and try, today, to listen more (than fifty percent) of the time? **#Habit**

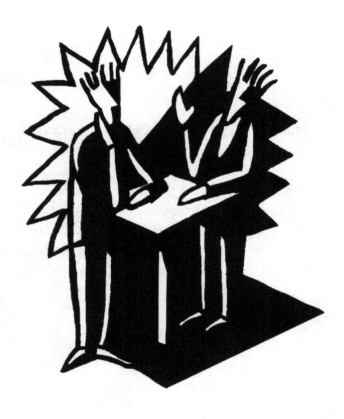

KINDNESS

☾

Humanitas: Humanity, Culture, Courtesy, Philanthropy, **Kindness.**

In order to receive, you must firstly give. Sustained joy and happiness comes from your contribution to another. Kind words can be short and easy to speak, but their echoes are both endless and timeless. Consider how, today, you can serve another? **#Habit**

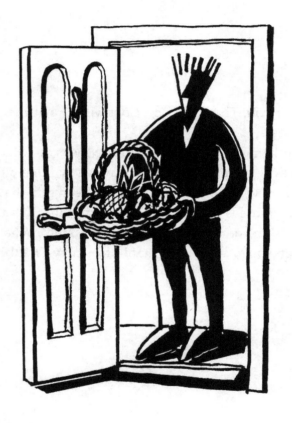

GRATITUDE

Gratia: Thanks, Grace, Goodwill, **Gratitude.**

When we make a daily effort to focus on what we are grateful for, studies have shown that our positive feelings increase. It has been said that very little is needed to make a happy life; it is all within yourself in your way of thinking[2]. What can you give heartfelt thanks for today? **#Habit**

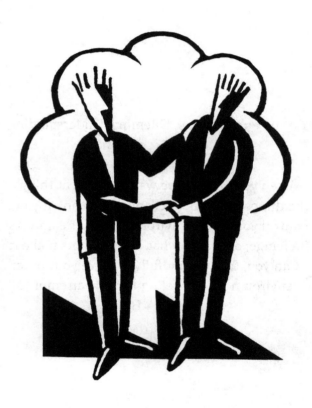

PERCEPTION

Comprensio: Scope, Dilemma, Understanding, Idea, **Perception.**

When you change the way you look at things, the things you look at change[1].You can only ever control your inner environment, as the universe *is* change; our life is what our thoughts make it[2]. Can you, today, mindfully observe your outer environment and relinquish any attempt to control? **#Habit**

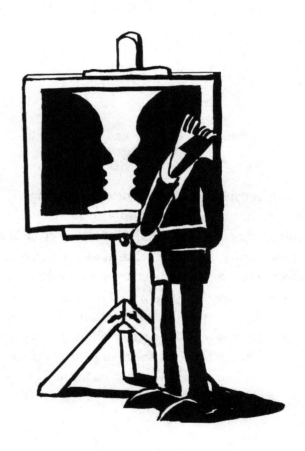

JOURNAL

Diurnus: Daily, Lasting a Day, Writing,
Journal.

By setting aside a notebook and finding a minute or two to write a sentence about the first thing that comes to mind, the brain is given the opportunity to unload some of its cargo. Think of a full box of chocolates: if you wanted to put a new chocolate in, you would have to remove one first. Why not write down one thing you give thanks for and see what follows? Can you, today, begin to create space in your mind and journal a few words? **#Habit**

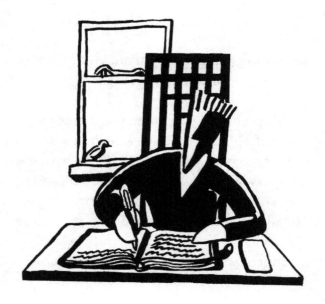

JUDGEMENT

Sententia: Sentence, Opinion, View, Decision, Thought, **Judgement.**

When you judge another, you define only yourself; yet each time you send best wishes in response to hate, you diffuse it. Some have made progress by 'faking until they make it', and we all know that practice makes perfect. When today you feel yourself about to judge, pause and ask yourself: can you instead send understanding and compassion? **#Habit**.

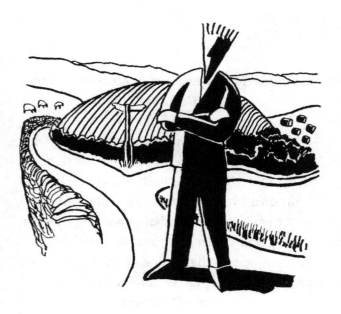

TOLERANCE

Indulgentia: Patience, Endurance, Resistance to Judge or Criticise, **Tolerance**.

Acknowledging that we each have our own journey to travel and that there is no right or wrong direction allows each of us to be present in our own lives. We can never truly control our outer environment or that of another; we can only ever control our own personal inner environment. What action or environment of another can you, today, tolerate with an open mind? **#Habit**

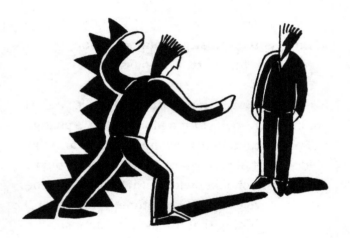

COMPASSION

Compassio: Sympathy, Commiseration, Mercy, Humanity, **Compassion.**

To move forward, you must first forgive yourself or another; so, just for a moment, try a change of perception. Replace condemnation and the judgement of yourself or another with a bid to understand or acknowledge that each of us does the best we can at any one time. What grudge are you hiding that, today, you can instead consider through a lens of mercy and compassion? #**Habit**

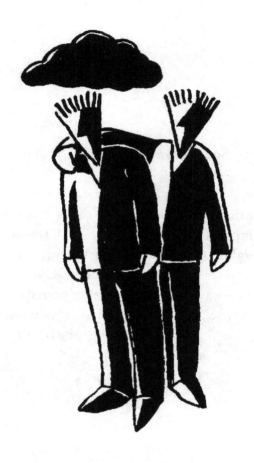

PAIN

Delor: Sorrow, Grief, Heartache, Twinge, **Pain.**

This is caused by intense or damaging stimuli arising from loss. At these times, it is really important to be kind to yourself (through thoughts, actions, and nourishment) and try to surrender (allowing the feelings to wash over you like waves). What you resist persists, and so ask yourself: what, today, can you stop resisting and instead surrender to? **#Habit**

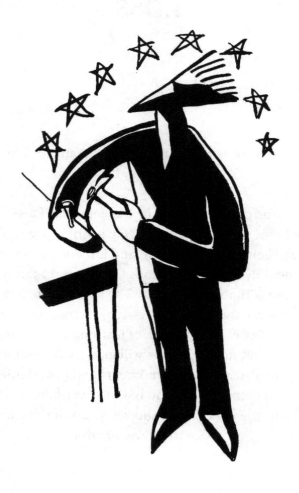

LOSS

Detrimtentum: Damage, Detriment, Waste, Defeat, Grief, **Loss.**

Grief can be invoked by many forms of loss, whether it be that of a job, a person, a marriage, or health, to name a few, and is a normal—and notably healthy—response, but unfortunately one without a timetable. The stages of denial, anger, bargaining, depression, and acceptance are all part a framework of learning to live with loss, but no two people will grieve in the same way. Pause for a few moments and consider if there is a loss you have not yet fully acknowledged and/or allowed yourself time and space to grieve. **#Habit**

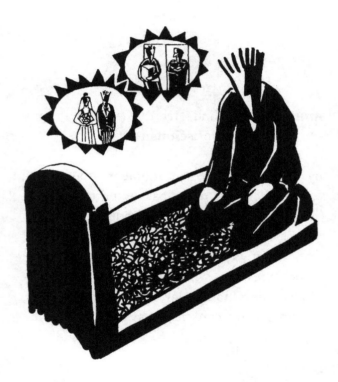

CONSCIOUSNESS

Animus: Soul, Mind, Heart, Affections, Purpose, **Consciousness.**

By observing the present moment—the here and now—the regret of the past and the fear of the future often fall away. Mindfulness and conscious action dissipate anxiety and feelings of negativity. It has been said that the soul becomes dyed with colour of its thoughts[2]. What one action, today, can you pause, focus, and become consciously aware of? **#Habit**

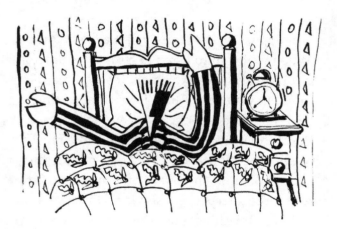

PEACE

Pax: Goodwill, Calmness, Quiet, Lull, **Peace.**

Finding peace is a journey, not a destination. When we begin to listen to a song, we are not simply waiting for it to finish. If each breath is a note in your song, then, from time-to-time, perhaps acknowledge that your next breath, whilst expected, is not guaranteed. We breathe twenty-five thousand times a day, taking thirty pounds of air in and out of our lungs, and how we breathe affects every single bodily system we have. Breathing more slowly might seem counterintuitive, but, by taking fewer breaths per minute, you can drastically improve your oxygen efficiency. Obesity, anxiety, depression, and poor digestion are some of the conditions breathing well has been shown to improve. Can you, today, observe five or ten of your breaths?
#Habit

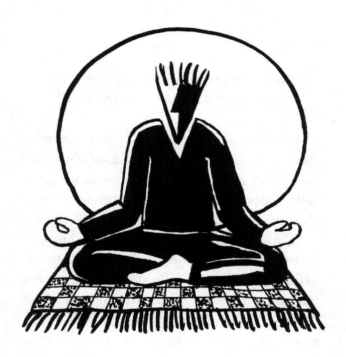

TECHNOLOGY

Nulla: Process, Reach, Equipment, TV, Smartphone, Tablet, **Technology.**

It has been reported that our attention span has been reduced to below that of a goldfish; our senses are regularly overloaded with nudges, notifications, and alerts. With the emission of blue light, our sleep has become eroded by the tech around us; our brains are becoming confused as to whether the body needs to be alerted or slowed down for sleep. TVs don't rest our mind, but simply pause the mind until the TV is switched off. By observing your evening screen time and switching your smartphone to airplane mode an hour before you want to be asleep, you will be amazed by the return to restorative sleep. Can you try, today, a tactical evening tech break? **#Habit**

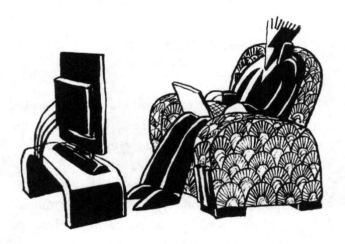

WATER

Unda: Wave, Ripple, Stream, Fluid, Liquid, **Water.**

Our brains, lungs, hearts, and kidneys are made up of more than seventy percent water. Stagnant water is poisonous; running water remains clear and clean, and we need fresh water to survive. Dehydration lowers mood, causes headaches, constipation, and much worse. As your brain is strongly influenced by your hydration status, up your intake of water to two litres per day. Can you, today, create a habit to drink more (pure) water? **#Habit.**

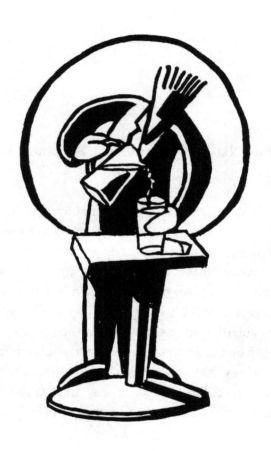

FOOD

☾

Cibus: Nutrient, Nourishment, Structural, Keep, **Food.**

Your body is the structure that carries you around, and food is the fuel it needs to keep the engine revving. Is your body a prestige supercar or a rusty three-wheeler spluttering old banger? Note and take to heart that the mind and body are inextricably linked. In 2003, the World Health Organisation began the five-day campaign to encourage people to eat fresh fruit and veg. Are you putting quality fuel in your engine daily? Can you, today, maximise the quality of the fuel you are putting in your body? **#Habit**

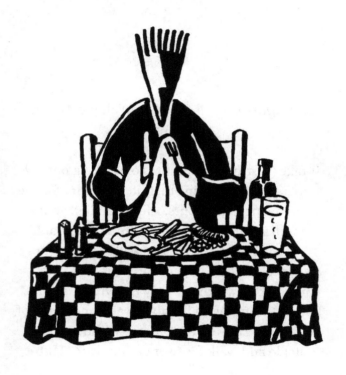

WALKING

Ambulatio: Stroll, Ramble, Walking About, **Walk.**

It takes just twenty minutes of walking outside to increase endorphins that lift positivity for the following eight hours. After walking, your mood/attitude are quickly lifted (and should your berating voice resist walking alone in silence, tell it to be quiet!). There is no such thing as bad weather—only the wrong clothes. Twilight brings with it unbelievable moments of stillness. How early, tomorrow, can you get outside and walk for twenty minutes? **#Habit**

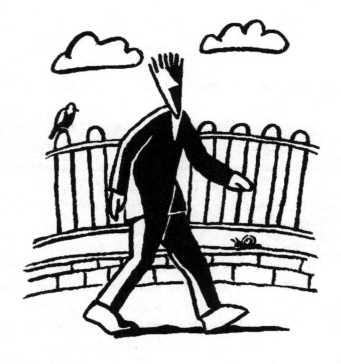

NATURE

Natura: Universe, Element, World, **Nature.**

In creation, plants and trees start out as tender and fragile, yet succeed in withstanding brutal wind, rain, and storms. Suppleness and softness are attributes of life, whereas hardness and brittleness are muses of death. Nature has a time and place for all things, and so the next time you feel strained, angry, anxious, and/or lost, go for a walk in nature and look around you and see the miracle of which you are a part. Chaos often exists in nature, and it has been said that nothing happens to anybody who is not fit to bear it[2]. Will you, today, be an impatient fool, or can you progress softly with deliberate discipline and patience? **#Habit**

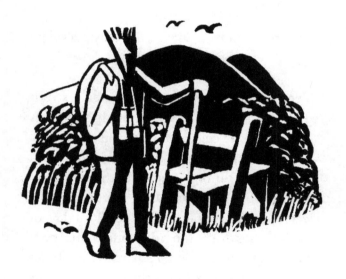

EVENINGS

Vespere: Even Fall, Sunset, Sundown, Twilight, Nightfall, **Evening.**

Sleep and the circadian system exert a strong regulatory influence on the immune system. It is all about the cells, and sleep has a specific function and role linked to immunology memory. Our bodies need both sufficient quantity and quality of sleep—but restorative sleep does not happen by accident! All day, our mind's senses are bombarded, and so our bodies need sleep to reset and recharge. The phrase 'circadian rhythm' infers the body's need for consistent routines. Establishing and then maintaining a regular evening routine will open your eyes to a whole new world of shuteye and restful sleep. What preparation for sleep can you start tonight? **#Habit**

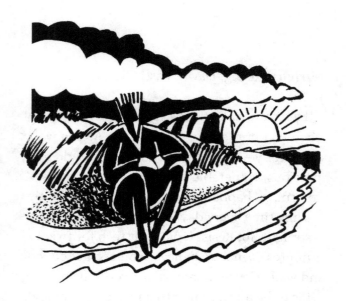

MORNINGS

Oriens: Rising, Dawn, East, Orient, **Morning.**

If you can make time to get the day on-track, then you start ahead of the game. As you wake, treat your mind gently like you would a precious, vulnerable seedling. The best possible mornings happen when an alarm is set for the same time every day; no dozing, just getting straight up. Resist looking at tech for twenty minutes or more whenever you can get outside and walk. Contemplate what a precious privilege it is to be alive; to breathe; to think; to enjoy[2]. Can you tonight set an alarm tonight for tomorrow (and the rest of the week) twenty-five minutes earlier than today, and get up and go outside to embrace the fresh start of a brand new day? **#Habit**

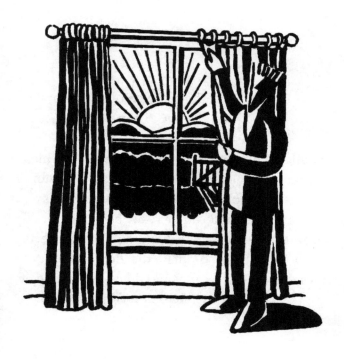

CAFFEINE

Julius: Drug, Central Nervous System, Stimulate, **Caffeine.**

Caffeine blocks the adenosine receptor (which initiates sleep) and will remain in the body for at least five hours after ingestion. Caffeine is a stimulant and can be really bad news for someone with anxiety. Caffeine's jittery effects on your body stimulate the 'fight or flight' response. Today, can you reduce your intake of coffee (or switch to decaf)? **#Habit**

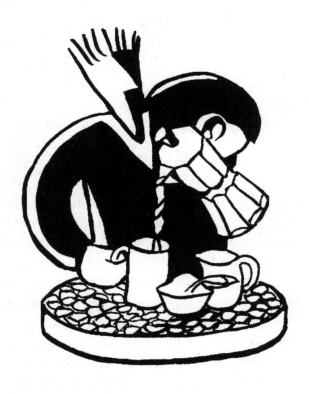

ALCOHOL

Volcatus: Liquor, Booze, Spirits, **Alcohol.**

The health warnings of this social norm are largely hidden and/or ignored. Put bluntly, it is a glass full of sugar which messes around with sleep, weight, and mindset. Fuel, water, and oil are the only liquids you put in your car, and less conspicuous of the physical downside of alcohol is its impact on positive mindset. Post-drinking (hours or even days later), alcohol is, at best, a negative influence—and at worst, it is a depressive catalyst. Can you try a 'tactical break' of three or more days and then observe any subsequent physical upsides and improved mindset? **#Habit**

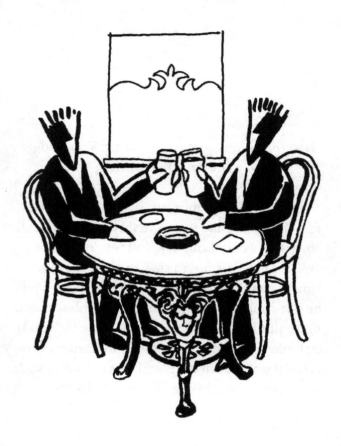

DISCIPLINE

Disciplina: Instruction, Training, Knowledge, Tuition, **Discipline.**

You are probably diligent in keeping your car full of fuel, oil, and water. In fact, if the fuel, oil, or water were to run dry, you would no doubt expect your car not to start or to break down. How much time does a man save each day when he does not look to see what his neighbour says, does, thinks[2]? Can you, today, keep your (good) fuel filled up, hydration high (a minimum of two litres of water each day), and fill your mind with good thoughts and feelings? **#Habit**

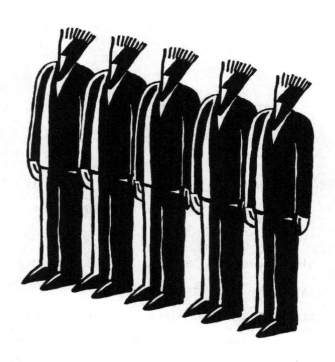

SHAME

Verecundices: Difference, Revenge, Bashfulness, **Shame.**

This small and innocent five-letter word plays a significant role in everyone's struggles. It is toxic, and must be faced courageously rather than silenced and shouted down. First, forgive yourself: before you step into the future, you must release the shackles of the past. It has been observed that it is not the snakebite that kills a man, but rather the venom that continues to flow through his veins[1]. What, today, can you forgive yourself for? **#Habit**

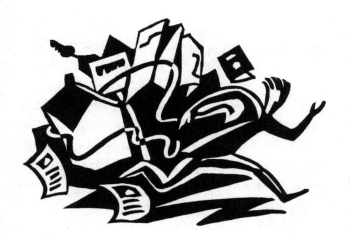

DREAM

Somnium: Fancy, Rave, Form of Planning, Self-Belief, **Dream.**

Without leaps of the imagination or dreaming, we lose the excitement of possibilities. There is one thing that makes a dream impossible to achieve, and that is the fear of failure. Stop, pause, take a deep breath, and then ponder for a few minutes: what dream can you blissfully contemplate today? **#Habit.**

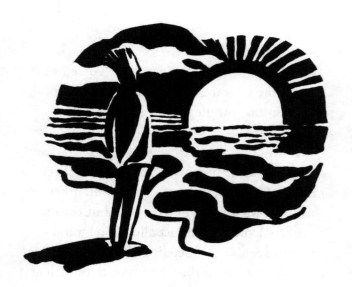

EGO

Ego: False Self, the Imagination, Voice in the Head which Berates, Obsession with Fear of the Future and Regret of the Past, **Ego.**

Have you noticed that, when you are tired and anxious (and/or hungover), the berating voice is rampant? If you can take a quiet walk in nature, just observe instead of trying to shut the voice down. Don't resist; just allow. The mind is always speaking of needless drama, wants, or worries. The ego of the mind tries to punish and detach from the inner self—that is, the heart and gut. When the ego has quietened, peace evolves. How much time today can you sit or walk alone and find a few moments of absolute peace and quiet? **#Habit**

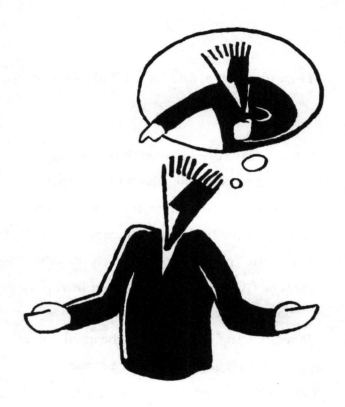

ALIGNMENT

Trutinor: Weigh, Balance of Mind and Body, **Alignment.**

When you have questioned the voice (ego) in your mind and have alignment to your true self, you will have the balance of thought, where optimism and hope can, with contentment, dominate. The focus is often solely on either 'emotional happiness' or 'physical fitness'. If the body is not aligned, the mind will have difficulty; and, likewise, when the mind is not aligned, the physical body will be hindered. Can you observe a moment when, today, both your mind *and* body are given the optimal environment to thrive? **#Habit**

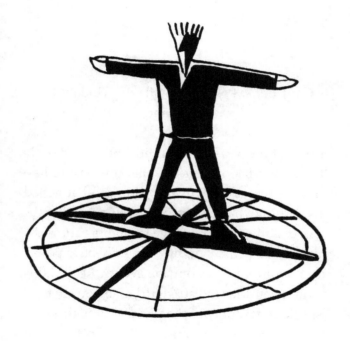

OPTIMISM

Confidens: Positive, Confident, Undaunted, **Optimism.**

Think of the '*yeses*' in your life and side-step the '*nos*'. It has been suggested that it is best to have a mind that is open to everything and attached to nothing; that no person knows enough to be a pessimist[1]. The negative thoughts can, with practice, just 'pass on by'. You only have power over your mind, not outside events. Realise this, and you will find strength[2]. Can you try to speak, today, only of the positive thoughts that come into your mind? **#Habit**

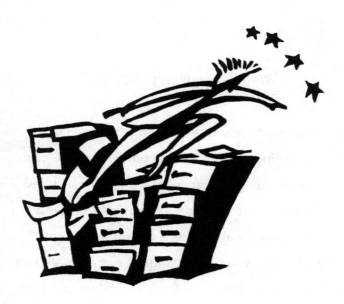

SMILE

Ridere: Laughter, Laugh, **Smile.**

Meet others with a smile, for the smile is the beginning and is so often contagious. The next mirror you pass, pause for a few moments and smile into it. How good does that feel? Death smiles at us all, but all a man can do is smile back+. Can you, today, smile at more (or all) you meet, and count how many seconds it takes for them to smile back? **#Habit**

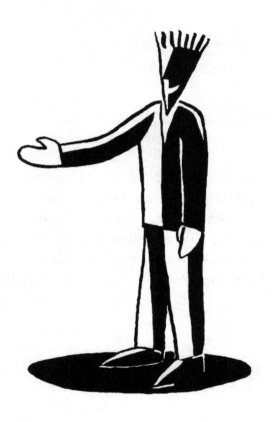

SELF-ACCEPTANCE

Sui Acceptatio: Approval, Accepting of Self-Asserting, **Self-Acceptance.**

It is not what others think or expect that is relevant, but how much you believe in yourself. It has been said that very little is needed to make a happy life; it is all within yourself in your way of thinking[2]. Who, today, do you acknowledge yourself to actually be? **#Habit.**

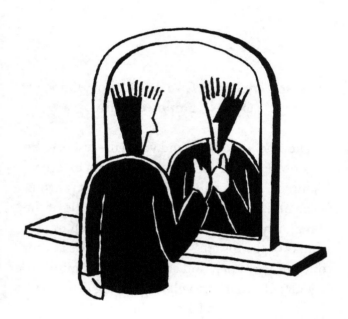

EMPOWERMENT

☾

Potestatem Facio: Give, Permission, Empower Oneself, **Empowerment.**

Believe you can do it and you will—excuses be gone[1]. Pleasure is often sought from external sources, but joy ultimately comes from within. The object of life is not to be on the side of the majority, but to escape finding oneself in the ranks of the insane[2]. Accept you are the author of your own story, and so, with that in mind, ask yourself: what role will the leading actor play today? #**Habit.**

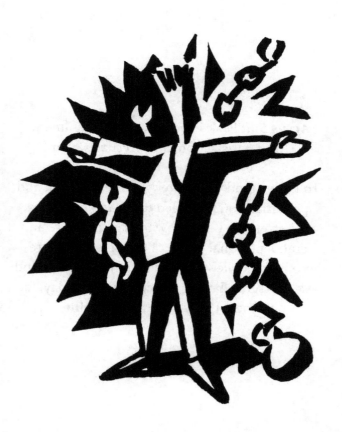

SELF-ACTUALISATION

☾

Actus Sui: Peak Experience, Self-Fulfilment, Grow, Satisfaction, **Self-Actualisation.**

To understand your inner greatness, talent, and potential, you first need to get to know your core strength. Learn how to stay in-centre and craft a personal vision of the person you are becoming. Review your habits, make a plan, and ask yourself: what do *you* commit to, today, for the next thirty-two days? **#Habit.**

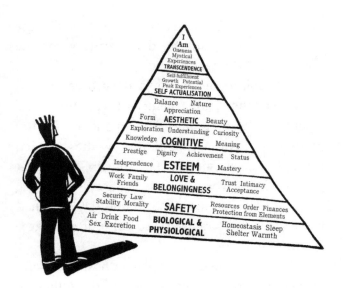

AND THEN...

O N THE THIRTY-THIRD NIGHT, the man lay in the dark, waiting for the lighthouse.

He took in several long, deep breaths, and reminisced how, only a month ago, he would resentfully tumble into bed, agitated, further increasing his own agitation as he scrolled through social media, peering in on other people's lives. Now, as he lay peacefully, feeling gratitude for various parts of the day that had passed, his body relaxed and calm, it felt like a lifetime ago.

The man's heart felt open with warmth, and he was proud of himself for the discipline he had undertaken with his new daily tasks. For weeks now, he had started the day calm and optimistic after eight hours of restorative sleep, which he was seeing to be as a result of consistently repeating his morning and evening routines. The man acknowledged that everything he had previously seen as pain was, indeed, a lesson, and that every other person in the world simply lived their lives, doing what they thought was their best at any one time. Finally, the man had got out of the bad #Habit of comparing himself to others.

He realised that by changing the way he thought about life, other people, and events, his resentment and excuses were gone. He was relieved that, finally, he was not afraid of showing affection or openly loving his family and close friends. He also felt overwhelming gratitude for his body and all it did: his lungs that gave him his every breath; his liver and kidneys that regulated his hormones, digestion, and waste; his eyes that allowed him to see the wonder of nature on his morning walks; his ears that allowed him to hear the birds singing at dawn; his nose that brought the fresh, fragrant, cool forest air. He felt wonderful—almost rebirthed—and, these days, he appreciated the nutritious food he ate that was thoughtfully selected with the intention to fuel his body. The daily two litres of water seemed to have stopped the headaches and brain fog he had so often experienced, and he once again felt alive.

Now, it felt like he belonged in his world. He felt connected and like he was a part of it, and he could see he was loved by those he cared about and that he was liked by the people he interacted with. The man now saw that, by giving first rather than waiting to receive, along with listening to others, many relationships in his life had been transformed. He was proud of his achievements over the past thirty-two days, and was curious to keep learning and aligning his body and mind further. He appreciated the beauty of all that Mother Earth provided; often, he would pause and look up towards the sky. Now, every night, he noticed the moon changing shape daily, as well as individual stars twinkling in the sky. Walking outside in the fresh air had become an important and enjoyable start to his day. He finally saw the future as exciting, and was beginning to feel fulfilled with what life held in the here and now. He no longer wanted more; he was truly grateful for all that he had and all that he was.

As the man drifted off to sleep on the thirty-third night, the lighthouse did not appear. The lighthouse's job was complete: another human being had understood that life takes effort, discipline, and good habits to nudge, motivate, and encourage a person to live the very best version of themselves and to be grateful for their relatively short existence on earth.

The man had wallowed in self-pity for so long that he had been unable to find any strength or impetus for action, but the man had seen the cycle he had been in: a lack of energy and enthusiasm to take action, meaning no action to make progress or heighten energy and enthusiasm.

The lighthouse had moved the man to celebrate his life and be truly grateful for everything he had achieved and every person he had provided and cared for. The man felt proud—proud to have lived the life he had, where lessons had been learned from pain, sent to him to forge and pursue, and allowed his greatness to shine through. These habits pieced together like a jigsaw, like bricks building a house, and had showed him a life that held hope, peace, and fulfilment—a life worth consciously living for and actively celebrating.

#Habit #Discipline #Perception #Gratitude #SelfActualisation

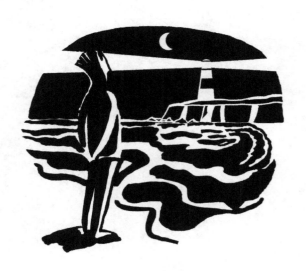

THE END

(

FURTHER RESOURCES

Set yourself up for success going forward with positively uplifting videos, habit tips and more, by joining us on social media:

f /Mandemic

in /in/NatashaJones

y /MandemicBook

○ /MandemicBook

Claim your FREE Positive Habits Sample Schedule so that you can take your first steps to forge your new pathway:

www.mandemic.co.uk

AUTHOR'S NOTE

MY LAST WORDS ARE to sing from the rooftops that self-care is absolutely crucial to having a spring in your step and functioning happily around hitting forty and beyond. A bit like the pictures in fairy tales of a stork delivering a baby, I believe that contentment in midlife does not just 'happen'; if self-care can be perceived as a discipline, not an indulgence, then the required determination and prioritisation becomes an accepted (and satisfying) way of life. Put simply, what work you put in will pay dividends in terms of wellbeing.

So many articles and books deal with either the mind *or* the body, but the two surely go hand-in-hand. To address one without the other is like saying you find Eric Morecambe funny but not Ernie Wise, or seeing Ant on TV but not Dec! Respect for yourself and who you choose to spend your time with is a simple place to start. Examples of actual self-care (rather than spa appointments, expensive chocolates, new bedding, etc.) could be:

- Saying 'no' to the thing you don't want to do, even if someone will be angry with you as a result.
- Stop watching Netflix, even though the next episode of the great series you have started to watch is already loading, because your alarm is going off at five so you can get to the gym or go for a walk/run before work.
- Letting others take care of themselves.
- Giving regular attention and thought to what food and liquids you do and do not put into your body.
- Declining the second drink at a social gathering—and sometimes even declining the first drink, full stop.

The late Dr Wayne W Dyer, who wrote more than two dozen books, compared the inside of a person to an orange: if you squeeze an orange, you can only get out orange juice (not lime, mango, or grapefruit juice); so, with this in mind, if a person has no love, care, or respect for themselves, how can they offer it to another?

How many divorces could have been avoided, the children then having one home rather than two, if Mum, Dad, or both had taken time to focus on their own self-care, rather than laying their misery and blame at their spouse's door?

It is, of course, your life, your choice, your chance at happiness, your body, and your decision whether to live the very best version of yourself (and leave others to live their lives), or do what you have always done and get what you have always got. Remember: if you want something to change, what you're doing (or not doing) has to change—and the place to start is in *your* inner world. Please do not ever forget that you *do* deserve the very best.

Perhaps pause, be quiet, and think for just a few moments.

**#Ego #Consciousness #Dream
#SelfActualisation**

WITH GRATITUDE

Throughout this book, I have made reference to a number of widely used statements, philosophies and ideals. I have found these to be incredibly valuable and perspective-changing, and they have allowed me to further reinforce and emphasise the points and habits. Most notably, where referenced, these refer to:

[1] Dr Wayne W Dyer; and
[2] Marcus Aurelius.

Moreover, I have been, and continue to be, inspired by the following, all of whom can be found in various resources and on various mediums, including books, podcasts, eBooks, YouTube, Google, and more. To all of you: I am thankful for your appearance into my life. Your timing was just perfect. **#Gratitude**

Lao Zu

Jean Pierre Weill

Eckhard Toille

Paul Coelo

Robin Sharma

Dr Rangan Chatterjee

Andy Ramage

Genevieve Davies

Helen Schucman

Simon Hass

Esther and Jerry Hicks

Owen Kane

Russel Brand

Jay Shetty

Tony Robbins

Jim Rohn

Mary Kate Fallon

Stuart Pilkington

Olivia Stefanino

Chris Evans

Matt Rudd

Jordan Peterson

Matt Haig

Stuart Robinson

Susan Jeffries

CPSIA information can be obtained
at www.ICGtesting.com
Printed in the USA
LVHW081558150321
681577LV00010B/686

9 781913 206567